DRUGS AND SPORTS

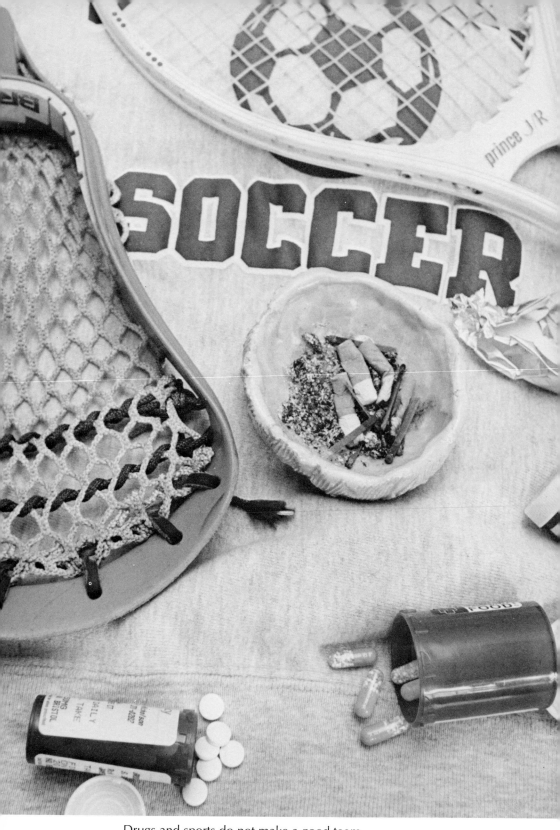

Drugs and sports do not make a good team.

THE DRUG ABUSE PREVENTION LIBRARY

DRUGS AND SPORTS

Rodney G. Peck

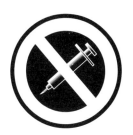

THE ROSEN PUBLISHING GROUP, INC.
NEW YORK

The people pictured in this book are only models; they, in no way, practice or endorse the activities illustrated. Captions serve only to explain the subjects of photographs and do not in any way imply a connection between the real-life models and the staged situations.

Published in 1992 by The Rosen Publishing Group, Inc.
29 East 21st Street, New York, NY 10010

First Edition

Manufactured in the United States of America.

Library of Congress Cataloging-in-Publication Data

Peck, Rodney G.
    Drugs and sports / Rodney Peck. — 1st ed.
    (The Drug Abuse Prevention Library)
    Includes bibliographical references and index.
    Summary: Discusses why athletes use different drugs, how they become addicted, the consequences of drug abuse, and how to get help.
        ISBN 0-8239-1420-8
        1. Doping in sports—Juvenile literature.
        2. Anabolic steroids—Health aspects—Juvenile literature. [1. Athletes—Drug use. 2. Drug abuse.] I. Title. II. Series.
        RC1230.P43 1992
        362.29'08'8976—dc20   92-12359
                                     CIP
                                     AC

Contents

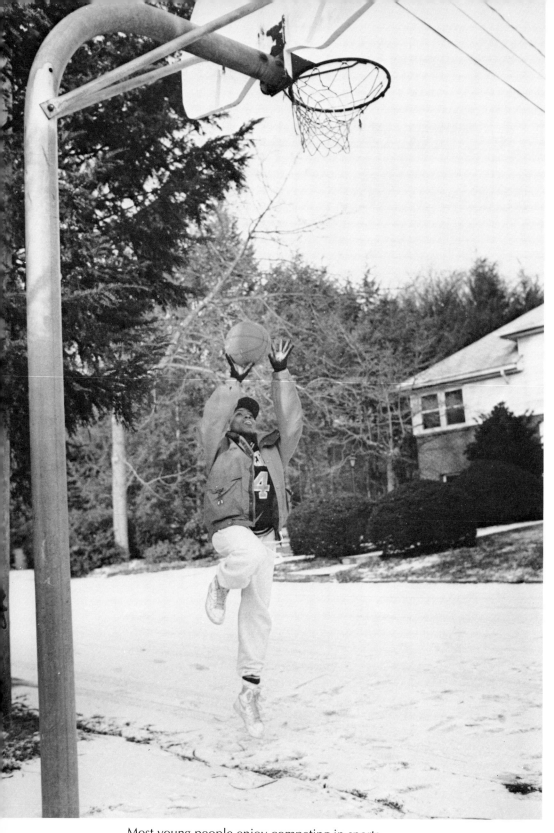

Most young people enjoy competing in sports.

CHAPTER 1

What Is Drug Addiction?

*E*very day in the United States kids are playing sports. It doesn't matter if it's winter or summer or indoors or outdoors. It doesn't even matter if the sports are well organized or not. Playing sports is fun, and somewhere today some young people are getting together to take part in a sport.

Somewhere today young people are also using drugs. It doesn't matter if it's summer or winter for drugs either. In this book you will read about sports and about drugs. You will learn why the two do not go together. The information is for you to think about and for you to discuss with friends and family.

8   First you need to know certain things about drugs and drug abuse. Some questions need to be answered. What is considered a drug? What drugs do people usually start with? How do people become involved with drugs? What is drug abuse? How do people become addicted?

What Is Considered a Drug?

It is very important to know which drugs you should be taking and which you should not be taking. Of course, it is okay to take medicine that a doctor or your parents give you for an illness. It is not okay to take medicine given to someone else, even if both of you have the same illness. Each prescription is different. What is okay for one person might hurt you.

What about other drugs? Most of us know that marijuana is a drug. We also know that cocaine and crack are drugs. But did you know that alcohol is a drug? Beer, wine, liquor, and wine coolers are all drugs. Tobacco is a drug, too. Cigarettes are made of tobacco. They have harmful effects on your health. We will deal with those drugs later. For now just remember that alcohol and tobacco are drugs as well as marijuana, cocaine, crack, and steroids.

What Is Drug Abuse?

Many people think that drug abuse is using a drug every day. Other people think that drug abuse is what they show on TV or in the movies—the wino who sleeps in the street or the prostitute who uses cocaine. But that is not always true.

A person can use a drug only once a week and still be a drug abuser. A person can use a drug once a month or once a year and still be a drug abuser. How is that possible?

It is possible because it does not matter how often the person gets drunk or high. What is important is what happens to him or her when drunk or high.

Does the person get angry more easily when drunk or high? Does the person ignore others or treat them badly? Is the person doing things that are not normal for him or her? If so, the person is abusing a drug. Most abusers mistreat themselves and others.

How Do People Become Addicted?

Most people who are drug addicts followed a pattern of drug use before they became addicted. So there is a process to becoming addicted to drugs. Addiction does not

10 happen overnight. No one wakes up one day and says, "I think I want to be a drug addict." *Nobody* takes drugs to become addicted. When people take their first drink, they don't do it because they want to become alcoholics. When people try their first cigarette they do not expect to get hooked. Drug use begins very innocently and then follows the pattern to addiction. The pattern goes like this:

1. Casual use/experimentation (body builds tolerance)

2. Regular use (body builds more tolerance)

3. Addiction or chemical dependence

A high school athlete named Patty will show you how she became addicted.

Casual use is the first step in drug addiction. Patty first took speed when she was 14. She thought, "A little upper can't hurt me." Some friends on the basketball team used it. Patty thought speed couldn't be bad for her. She only took it when someone gave it to her. She liked the way it made her feel. It also gave her more energy for basketball games.

Patty did not realize that whenever you put drugs into your body they change the way the body works. It does not matter

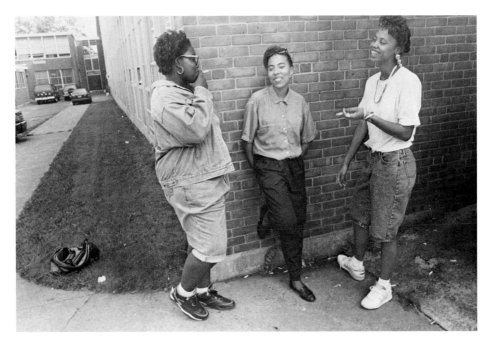

Cigarette smoking can lead to dependence on the drug nicotine.

what drug you use. The body changes even if you use only small amounts. Drugs cause negative changes in the body.

Tolerance slowly builds up toward drug addiction. Patty was taking speed only once in a while. But something happened in her body. Her body built up tolerance. It changed. It had become used to the speed. To get the same high, Patty needed to take more speed. Tolerance makes the body need more of the drug in order to get the same high.

The body builds tolerance to any drug. For example, let's say Patty drinks two wine coolers every Friday to get "buzzed." After a while Patty's body will say, "Sorry, two coolers won't do the job anymore." To

11

12 get the buzz she wants, Patty will have to drink three or four coolers. That is tolerance. The body also builds up tolerance to alcohol, tobacco, speed, cocaine, or any other drug.

Regular use is the next step in drug addiction. Eventually Patty started taking speed every day during the basketball season. It helped her get through practices and games. She was using speed on a regular basis. She wanted the high more and more often. She started finding people from whom she could buy speed. She still didn't think she had an addiction problem, though.

Addiction, the last step, is also called *chemical dependence.* The basketball season ended, but Patty continued taking speed. She took it to stay up and study at night. She took it before school to have energy for the day. She spent her lunch money on speed. She spent her allowance. Her enthusiasm for sports started to drop. She was tired much of the time. Even her social life was sad, but she didn't care. Patty needed speed just to feel normal. She depended on the chemicals in speed. She was addicted to it.

That is the process of addiction. There is one big difference between regular use

and addiction. When people are addicted |
they use the drug even when it causes bad things to happen in their lives.

Patty started out slowly. At first it was no big deal to take speed. But Patty did not count on her body's building tolerance to the drug. Teenagers like Patty need to be extremely careful with tolerance. In your teens your body is growing. Because the body is changing, it builds tolerance to drugs more easily.

A person who is 15 years old will become addicted to drugs 10 times faster than an adult. An adult might take 10 *years* to become an addict. A young person might take 10 *months*. Why? Because a young, growing body builds tolerance faster than a mature body. Then the person taking the drugs needs more to reach the same high.

Taking speed became a regular habit during basketball season. Patty told herself that she used it to get more energy. She was lying to herself. Her casual use had turned into regular use. When the season ended she did not stop using speed. She started using more. She was addicted. Her school work suffered. She didn't do things with her friends anymore. The drug became the most important thing to Patty. She used her allowance to buy

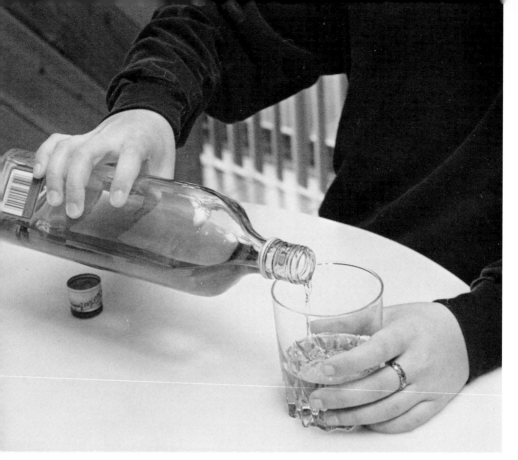

Feeling the need to drink alcohol every day may be a sign of addiction.

speed. If she had no money, she would steal from her mother's purse.

Any drug can lead to addiction. Alcohol and marijuana are drugs. Tobacco itself contains the drug nicotine. Cocaine, speed, and steroids are all drugs. People can become addicted to any of them. Don't let anyone tell you that one drug is safer than another.

Who Becomes Addicted?

Anyone can become addicted. Addiction happens to rich people and poor people. It happens to black, white, red, and yellow people. It happens to athletes. Yes, even people who are in the best physical shape are not safe from drug addiction.

People who have family members who are drug addicts or alcoholics need to be extra careful. Drug addiction and alcoholism are like some other diseases. The disease is easily passed from one generation to another.

Your family can often play a big part in whether you will use drugs. Being around drugs in your home affects the way you look at them. Parents who use drugs send a bad message that drugs are okay.

What Is Drug Addiction?

Now you know how a person can become addicted to drugs. But what really is drug addiction or chemical dependence? How do you know if someone has it?

This is very important for you to remember. *Drug addiction is a disease.* Like any disease, it has symptoms. People with the disease of addiction have an urge to use alcohol or other drugs. They use the drug even if it causes a lot of problems in their lives. That means that they are not in control of the disease. Addicted people have mood swings. They hang out with

16 | different crowds. They show their symptoms in the way they behave.

You should understand a few more things. A chemically dependent person does not use the drug because he wants to. He uses it because he needs to. Once a person has the disease, he cannot get rid of it. But he can control it—with help.

Where Does Addiction Begin?

As we have seen, drug abuse starts very innocently. It usually starts with something called a *gateway drug*.

Tobacco, alcohol, and marijuana are all gateway drugs. They are easy for young people to get. They are also the drugs that usually lead to the use of other drugs. When people drink alcohol or get high on pot for a while, they get bored and want to try something new. They think that they can easily get away with using alcohol or marijuana without having problems. Then they think that maybe steroids or cocaine or crack are not really as bad as people say they are.

Tobacco, alcohol, and marijuana are called gateway drugs because they open the gate for further drug use. People start with the gateway drugs and end up using harder ones.

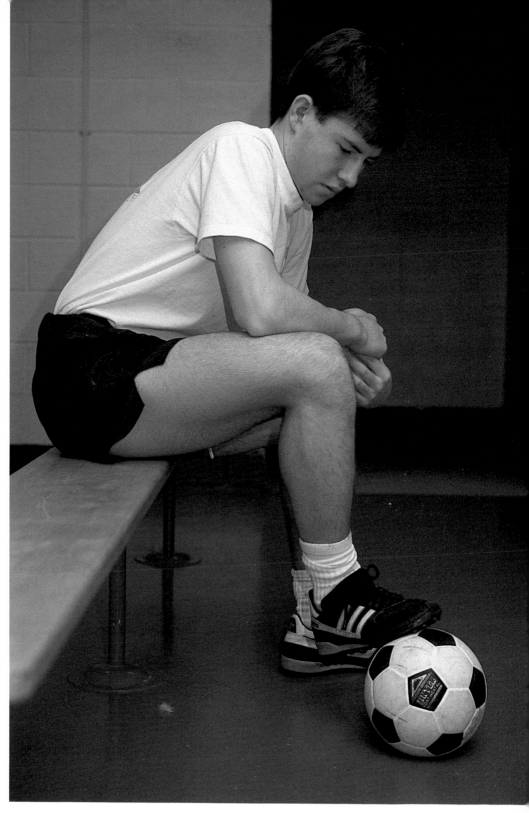

Loss of energy may be a symptom of a drug problem.

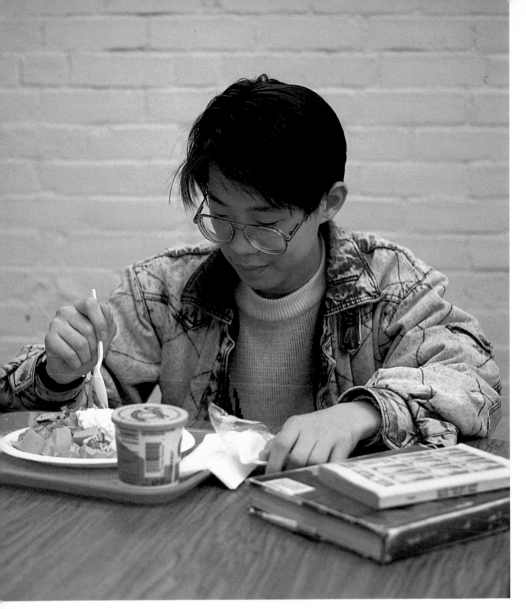

Everything you put into your body affects you. Healthful foods are important for keeping your body in top condition.

Experimentation

Drug use normally starts during the teen years. During that time there is a lot of pressure to do what your friends are doing. Let's check out a few examples of experimentation with gateway drugs.

Smoking Cigarettes

A friend sneaks a pack of cigarettes from his parents. You decide to smoke one. You think, "Why not?" You are "just experimenting." Cigarettes are no big deal, right? A lot of adults smoke. It must not really be all that bad for you. Wrong! Cigarettes are made of tobacco. Tobacco contains a very addictive drug called nicotine. It also contains a substance called tar. Cigarettes can cause lung cancer and other diseases.

Drinking Alcohol

The crowd is going to a party. It will be the best party of the year. But there will be alcohol. The pressure to drink will be strong. Some people will not be strong enough to say no. Some people will drink to see what it feels like to be drunk. They are just experimenting.

Smoking Marijuana

You're hanging out with a group of people. A couple of them are your good friends. The others are just from school. One of them pulls out a joint and lights it up. It is passed around, and everyone takes a "hit." You have to make a decision right on the spot. You don't want the pot, but you don't want to seem like a jerk.

20   Young people decide to "experiment" with gateway drugs for a lot of reasons:

- To forget their problems.
- To be cool.
- To seem older or mature.
- To rebel against their parents.
- To do what their friends do.
- To be popular.

Using drugs does not make problems go away. It only adds to the problems that already exist. Drugs do not make you cool either. Ask yourself, "What is cool about throwing up or passing out when you are drunk?" Also, being mature has nothing to do with drugs. Being mature means that you make healthy decisions for your life. Do things because you want to do them, not because your friends want you to. The decision should be yours.

People who use drugs to rebel think that it will hurt their parents. That is true. Taking drugs probably will hurt the parents. It also hurts the person who is taking the drugs. Taking drugs to rebel hurts everybody.

Peer pressure is a big problem to face. If you feel pressure to use gateway drugs, you will feel pressure to use other drugs, too. Don't give in to the pressure.

CHAPTER 2

Steroids

*S*teroids are the most abused drug in the history of athletics. They are used at every level of competition. Athletes of all ages are involved in steroid use. What are steroids? What do they do to you? How can you tell if someone you know is taking steroids?

Our bodies make natural chemicals called hormones. They are the chemicals that control how we grow. The hormone in boys and men is called *testosterone*. It mostly controls muscle growth and height. Testosterone controls all the things that turn boys into men.

22   Steroids are chemicals, too. But they are made in a laboratory. Steroids are fake testosterone in pill or liquid form. The liquid can be injected with a needle.

Taking steroids changes the way the body grows and functions. The human body is a perfect machine if it is treated well. The body knows how much sleep it needs and how much food it needs. The body also knows how much testosterone it needs for healthy growth. The extra testosterone from steroids only confuses the body. Then bad things can happen.

Someone taking steroids can look forward to a lot of problems. That includes boys *and* girls. People think that steroids will make them faster, bigger, and stronger. That may be true for a while, but it does not last. People taking steroids have problems with their health. They have problems thinking and acting normally. There are more bad points to taking steroids than good points.

Steroids are imitation testosterone. They can turn off your body's real hormone system. They can even cause you to stop growing. Dr. Robert O. Voy says, "If you take these drugs during adolescence you will turn off the body's normal mechanism for long-bone growth." That means that

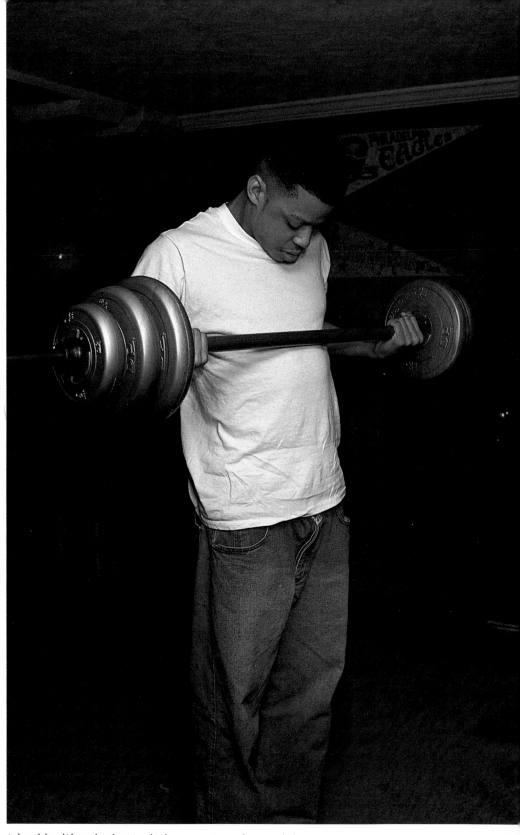

A healthy lifestyle that includes exercise, plenty of sleep, and a balanced diet is the best way to build a strong body.

24 you will not reach the height that your body is supposed to reach.

Many other changes take place, too. Most young people who use steroids get severe acne on the face, chest, back, and arms. Some people get bad headaches. Steroid users often have a high temperature. Some even get nosebleeds. Others lose their hair. All of these problems are small compared with the big damage that steroids can do.

The combination of steroids and the human body is deadly. Steroid users get a buildup of a fat called *cholesterol.* This fat clogs the arteries and veins. Blood cannot get through clogged vessels. The body has to work extra hard to push the blood through. That means the blood pressure goes up. Many steroid users end up with damaged hearts. Some of them even have heart attacks and die.

Remember that steroids turn off your body's hormone system? The hormone system is part of the reproductive system. The reproductive system is responsible for your sex glands. When your body's hormone system shuts down, so do the sex glands. Some young men find that their breasts get larger and their testicles shrink when they use steroids. Females who use

steroids may become sterile. They will not **25**
be able to have babies. They also grow
more hair on their bodies.

Another health problem with steroids is
cancer. In many users, tumors develop in
the liver, the kidneys, and the prostate.

As if that were not enough, there's
more. A nickname for steroids is "roids."
Something called "roid rage" is common
among steroid users. The increase in the
male hormone causes users to become
violent. Football players who have used
steroids say that roid rage made them
want to rip the heads off their opponents.
People who use steroids are often very
violent or aggressive off the field, too.
They are out of control and dangerous to
themselves and others. Serious mental
problems often result from steroid use.

So those are all the things that steroids
can give you. They can give you heart
attacks, tumors, acne, headaches, and so
on. They can also take things away from
you. People using steroids often lose their
memory. They lose their attention span.
They can't concentrate for very long. They
lose their ability to cope with stress. They
also lose their ability to feel pain.

Let's say that a runner pulls a muscle.
She takes a steroid injection so she won't

Drugs at a Glance

Alcohol: Alcohol can alter mood, cause changes in the body, and become habit-forming. Alcohol is a depressant. It slows the body down. It affects the central nervous system.

Signs of Use:
Bad judgment, loss of self-control and coordination, slow reactions, slurred speech, and sometimes blackouts.

Long-Term Effects:
Brain—Permanent cell damage, loss of memory, confusion.
Heart—High blood pressure, enlarged heart.
Liver—Swelling, cirrhosis.
Lungs—Swelling, chance of infection.
Sex Organs—Impotence.
Stomach—Ulcers.
Muscles—Weakness, loss of tissue.

Tobacco: Contains three dangerous chemicals: nicotine, tar, and carbon monoxide. Very addictive.

Signs of Use:
Shortness of breath, bad breath, coughing, asthma.

Long-Term Effects:
Blood—Creates high blood pressure.
Heart—Possible heart attack.
Lungs—Possible cancer, pneumonia, emphysema, bronchitis.
Mouth—Possible cancer.

Marijuana: Contains over 400 chemicals. Causes mood changes. Addictive.

Signs of Use:
Memory loss, loss of coordination, loss of concentration, loss of motivation, unusual fears.

Long-Term Effects:
Eyes—Redness.
Brain—Brain damage.
Heart—Low oxygen supply.
Lungs—Possible cancer.
Sex Organs—Damages normal sexual growth.

Cocaine: The most addictive drug. Changes brain chemistry.

Signs of Use:
Nosebleeds, loss of sleep, loss of weight, depression, violent behavior, the "shakes," loss of interest, poor appearance.

Long-Term Effects:
Central nervous system—Damage.
Brain—Permanent damage.
AIDS—Possible if cocaine is injected with an infected needle.
Heart—High rate, possible stroke or heart attack.

Crack: Powerful, smokable form of cocaine. Extremely addictive.

Steroids: Artificial male hormone. Dangerous to physical and mental growth.

Signs of Use:
Temporary increase in size, strength, and weight.

Long-Term Effects:
Brain—Drastic mood swings.
Blood—High blood pressure.
Kidney—Malfunction or failure.
Liver—Damage, possible tumor.
Skin—Tumors, acne.
Bone—Stops growth.
Sex Organs—Smaller testicles, infertility.

feel the pain. Then she runs. If she damages the muscle more, she won't feel it. She could destroy her running career by using the steroids and tearing a muscle.

The increasing number of people using steroids is costing a lot. The loss of health is a very high price to pay. So is the cost to those who start failing in school. The mental health of those people who often experience roid rage is also a serious cost.

The physical and mental costs are not the only problem. Steroids also cost money. Steroids are prescribed by some doctors, but most are bought illegally.

The price of illegal steroids depends on the dosage. The average cost for a steroid user is between $50 and $600 a month. People pay good money for steroids when all they get from them are problems.

Steroid use is the fastest growing drug epidemic. There are said to be 3 million users or more. Illegal sale of products is called the "black market." Right now, the black market in steroids is making $100 million every year. The people who sell steroids are getting rich by making other people sick. The pushers are the only people who benefit from steroids.

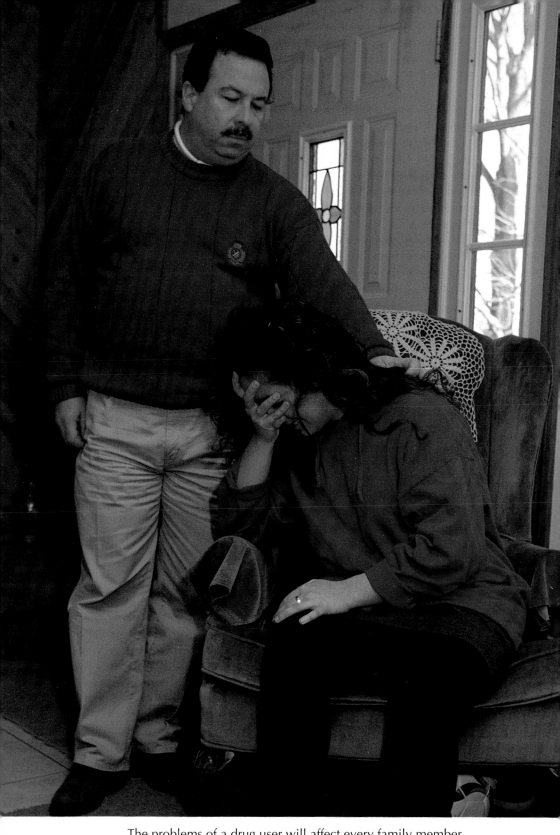

The problems of a drug user will affect every family member.

CHAPTER 3

Why Athletes Start Using Drugs

Some people start using drugs in middle school. Others start in high school. Why?

Peer Pressure

The most common reason that people use drugs is peer pressure. They start using drugs when their friends or teammates offer them some. Nobody wants to be called a "wimp" or a "goody-goody." Many people eventually give in. They think that if they don't use the drug the rest of the team won't like them.

That is called negative peer pressure. It is when you feel pressure to do something that you don't want to do. Negative peer

29

30 pressure is tough to face. Especially if you're facing a lot of people at once.

However, peer pressure does not have to be negative. Peer pressure can also be positive. Does your team have rules about drinking? About smoking or using other drugs? Those rules can be used for positive peer pressure. You can remind your teammates of the rules. You are not the only one who thinks that rules are a good idea. If your team does not have rules about drug use, maybe you could suggest having them. The rules need to state clearly the penalties for drug use. Talk to your coach or trainer.

There are other ways to use positive peer pressure. For example, don't go to parties where there will be alcohol or marijuana. Instead, throw a party of your own. Serve soft drinks or juices. Have rules about guests not coming drunk or stoned. That is a great way to boost positive peer pressure. It shows people that they do not need alcohol or other drugs to have fun.

If someone on your team is using drugs, try to encourage him or her not to use them. Be a positive role model. Try to get other team members to talk to the person. Tell the user that he is needed. Show your teammate that the team cares about him. Positive peer pressure is more powerful than negative peer pressure.

Negative peer pressure will always be around. Even when you are an adult you will face negative peer pressure to do some things. You need to decide, right now, how you will handle the pressure the next

31

Teens can be popular with friends by being drug-free and having a positive attitude.

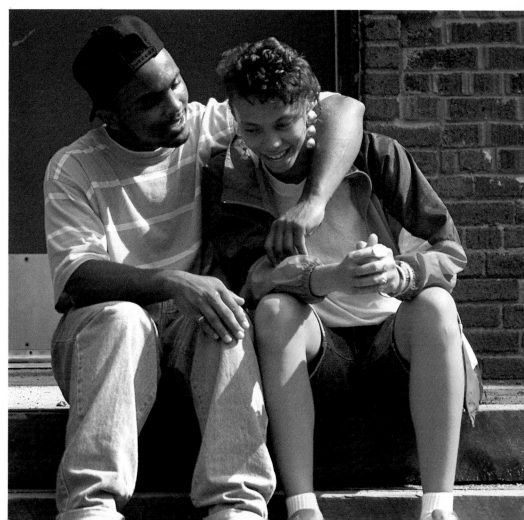

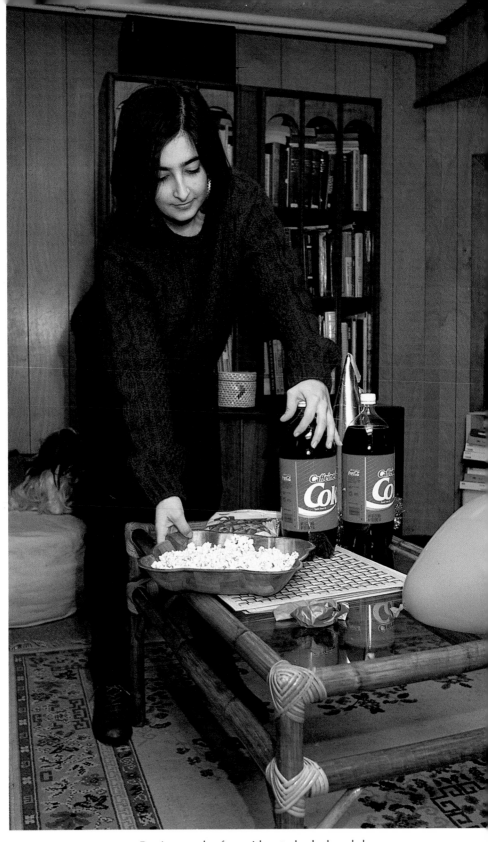

Parties can be fun without alcohol and drugs.

time. It's *your* body. It's *your* life. Don't
let other people persuade you to do bad
things with it. Be a positive example for
all the people around you.

To Be "Cool"

Bad things happen to people who use
drugs. They cause car accidents. They get
terrible health problems. They destroy
their families. They lose their jobs. They
get kicked off the team.

Yet many people still use drugs. Why?
Because they think, "It can't happen to
me," or "I won't get caught." They want to
prove that they can use drugs and be safe
from harm. They are wrong. Sooner or
later drug use will catch up with them.

Some people start using drugs to be
"cool." They drink alcohol to seem older
and more mature. They smoke pot or
snort cocaine because it is the trendy thing
to do. If the popular people are doing it,
others usually follow. They wrongly think
that using drugs will help them be accepted
by the popular group.

People become popular for many reasons.
Some are popular because they are smart.
Some are popular because they are talented
in music or drama. Others are popular
because they are student leaders.

34   Many people are popular because they play sports. Being an athlete carries a lot of responsibility. The athletes represent the school. They represent the other students, the teachers, and the whole town. It is important that they set a good example. They serve as role models for their peers and for younger people.

A responsible athlete is someone who thinks that being drug-free is cool. The only way to be popular and cool at the same time is to stay away from alcohol and other drugs.

To Look Good

Peer pressure to look good is another reason that athletes start using drugs.

Girls are expected to be thin. They are expected to have perfect breasts, flat stomachs, and slim hips. It's silly, but people think that is how ideal girls are supposed to be.

More and more young women are turning to drugs to try to achieve "the look." Thousands of women use diet pills (speed) to lose weight. Other young women have turned to steroids to build their bodies.

Young men are expected to look good, too. Guys are supposed to have hard, well-defined chests. They are supposed to have washboard stomachs and developed arms and legs. More and more young men also expect the use of drugs to help them get "the look."

35

It is important to look good and feel good about yourself. It is also important to know that you can change the way your body looks. But drugs will not do it for you. The only way to get the body you want is by hard work. You have to exercise and eat the right foods. A better body can only be achieved through determination and discipline.

Cleanliness and grooming make you look your best.

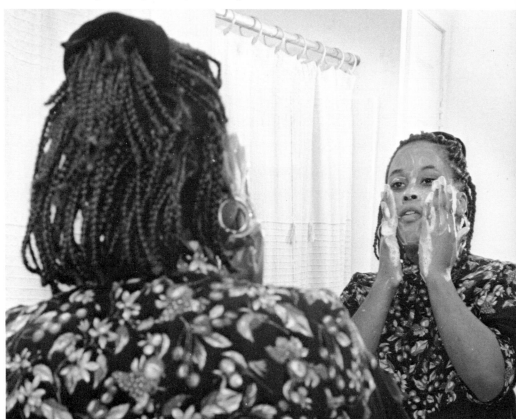

College Athletics

36

College athletes have some of the same problems that many younger athletes have. They feel pressure from some of their teammates to use drugs. They want to be accepted, too. There are some differences, however.

A lot of money is invested in college sports. A lot of money is also invested in college athletes. Most college athletes win full or partial scholarships to play sports for their school. Playing the sport is like having a job because the athletes get an education or money for it.

The coach of the team is like a boss. The athletes do what their boss tells them to do. Coaches usually want the best for their athletes. However, some coaches pressure their athletes to use drugs. A lot of money is involved. Some coaches will do whatever it takes to win, even if winning means that some players are using steroids or other drugs.

It is wrong for a person to use drugs. It is also very wrong for a coach to pressure an athlete to use drugs. Athletes must be very strong against drugs. No matter who offers the drugs, the answer should always be a firm no.

When one player uses drugs to compete, it starts problems for all the players.

For example, Joe plays for the Pigeons. He uses steroids to give him an edge over the other team's players. Bob plays for the Groundhogs. He finds out that Joe is using steroids. Bob knows that he won't be able to beat someone using steroids. So Bob thinks that he needs to take steroids just to be able to compete.

Some athletes do use drugs. Then other athletes use drugs to keep things even or "fair." But the only fair way to play is drug-free.

Professional Sports

Professional athletes are another story. Professional sports are big business. A lot of money can be made or lost. Professional athletes are paid large salaries. Having so much money makes it possible for them to afford drugs easily.

Pro athletes become famous. They start to feel that they can take on the world. Some get involved with drugs. Then they find that they are just like other people. They learn that drugs can destroy anybody, even star athletes.

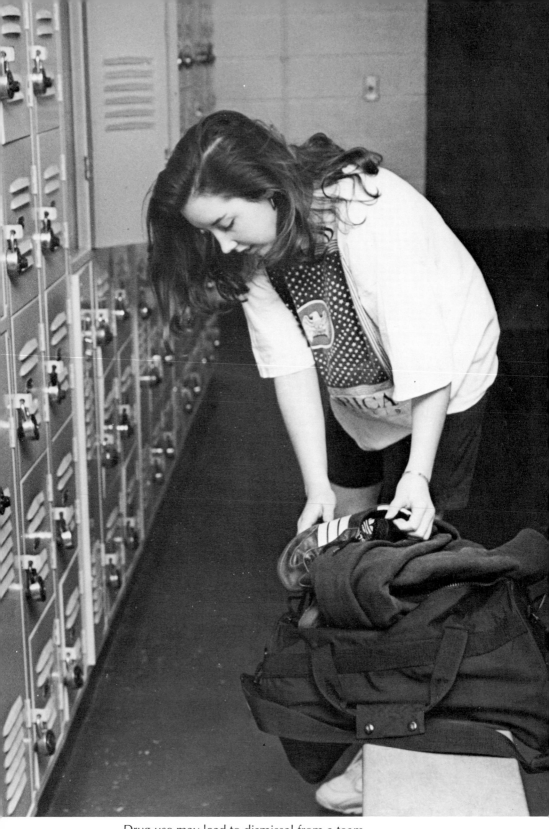

Drug use may lead to dismissal from a team.

CHAPTER 4

Athletes Who Chose Drugs

*I*t is important for us to learn from other people. We can learn a lot by watching their mistakes. Then we know how to avoid making the same mistakes.

Len Bias was a star basketball player for the University of Maryland. Professional teams from all over the country wanted him to play for them. In 1986, he was drafted to play for the Boston Celtics. Everything in his life seemed perfect. He was young. He was healthy. He had just been chosen to play for one of the best basketball teams in the world. There was a party in his honor. At the party, Len Bias

40 decided to use cocaine for the first or second time ever. He died of a heart attack soon afterward.

The sports world was shocked when Len Bias died. Still, some people did not learn the lesson about drugs.

The 1988 Summer Olympic Games were held in Seoul, Korea. Millions of people watched the Games on television. The very best athletes in the world competed.

Competition is always stiff in the track-and-field events. Fractions of a second make the difference between first place and last place in some events. The 100-meter dash is one of those events.

In the 100-meter, two of the athletes were Ben Johnson and Carl Lewis. They had raced each other many times, but this race would answer a question for the world: "Who is the fastest man alive?"

The starting gun went off. In a little less than 10 seconds, the race was over. Ben Johnson took first place. He broke the world's record. He was instantly known as the fastest man alive.

Then the sports world was shocked again. Drug testing was done. Ben Johnson admitted that he had used steroids. Using steroids is called cheating. The International Olympic Committee took away his gold medal and gave it to Carl Lewis.

Ben Johnson did not die from his drug use. But he had to suffer humiliation and shame. He had let down the entire country of Canada, which he represented. He lost the respect of other athletes. The entire world knew that he had cheated by taking drugs.

So much is lost when people use drugs. Len Bias lost his life. Ben Johnson lost a gold medal and a lot more. They are not the only athletes who have lost.

Steve Howe is a married man. He has two children. He used to play for the Los Angeles Dodgers in the early part of the 1980s.

In 1980, Steve was named Rookie of the Year. He was the best new professional player in his entire league. In 1981, Steve pitched in the World Series. The Dodgers won that year. In 1984, Steve was chosen to play in the All-Star game. He was having a very successful career. He had many good years to look forward to.

Then, Steve Howe used cocaine and his future changed. Cocaine became a big part of his life. He started having hallucinations (seeing things that were not there). Cocaine often causes hallucinations. Steve

42 would drive 150 miles just to buy more cocaine. He would leave his wife and not return for days at a time. His family and his career suffered greatly because he was using cocaine.

In 1984, Steve was suspended from baseball. He entered treatment programs five times. Each time he used drugs again. Addiction is very hard to fight. Once you start using drugs, it takes a long time to stop. Then you spend the rest of your life trying to stay off drugs. Steve has stopped using drugs now. That means he is a recovering drug addict. He learned the hard way what drugs can do.

Tony Anderson is another athlete who did not learn from other people's mistakes. He was a high school athlete in Valdosta, Georgia. He was on the varsity football team. The Valdosta Wildcats were the state champions 19 times. The people of Valdosta take their football seriously. They have great pride in their team. Tony Anderson was the star. They called him "Touchdown Tony." The best universities in the country offered him scholarships.

The Valdosta football team has a rule that athletes who use drugs are not allowed on the team.

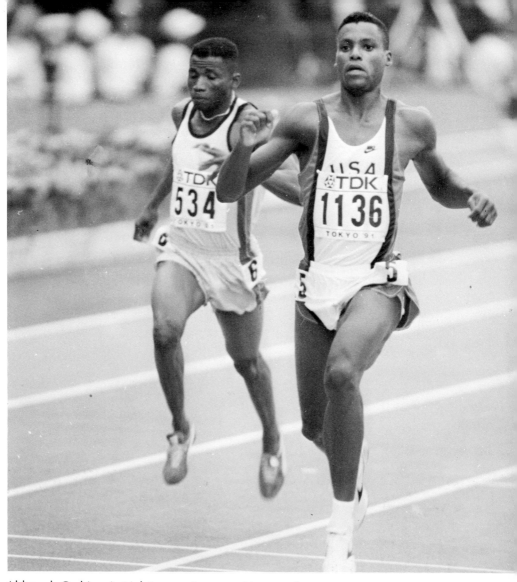

Although Carl Lewis (right) came in second in a track event at the 1988 Summer Olympics, he was given the gold medal that was taken away from Ben Johnson. Johnson had admitted taking steroids.

One day, Tony Anderson and some other players showed up drunk for a scrimmage game. The Valdosta coach stood by the rules. He kicked Tony Anderson, the star player, off the team. He also dismissed the other players who were drunk.

44

Tony's coach kicked him off the team because he was popular with the younger kids. When Tony was drunk at the game, he set a very bad example. The coach did not want the kids to think that drinking was okay. Tony was a good athlete, but he was not being a good role model.

Tony started using alcohol more often. Then he moved on to other drugs like marijuana and cocaine. One day, he was driving a car and hit someone. He thought the person was okay, so he drove away. Tony was arrested for reckless driving and for leaving the scene of an accident. He was released on 39 months' probation, but he had to check in with a probation officer regularly. Tony violated his probation. Now he is in prison. All his problems started when he decided to drink alcohol.

Len Bias, Ben Johnson, Steve Howe, and Tony Anderson are just a few of the athletes who have used drugs and lost. They learned the lesson too late.

What Else Is Lost?
Social Loss
Athletes hold a special place in the eyes of the community. They are highly respected because they have athletic talent.

Athletes are also role models. Young athletes look up to them. They want to be just as good when they get older.

When an athlete uses drugs, all that changes. Drug-using athletes lose the respect of people around them. No longer are they treated as special. The younger people no longer want to be like them.

What about the other players on the team? How do you think they treat a teammate who uses drugs? They think he is not too smart. They think that he ruined a good thing by using drugs. They have no respect for him at all.

People who use drugs also lose friends. Why? Because they start acting differently. They start treating people badly. Sometimes drug users are violent. Most people don't want to be around people who change when they use drugs.

Personality Loss

Drug-using athletes lose respect and friends. They say that they feel they have lost almost everything. Drugs make most athletes lose pride in themselves. These athletes usually feel that they have let everybody down.

Most of all, drug-using athletes lose the future. They will never know how good

46 they could have been or how far they could have gone. The world will never know if Len Bias would have been one of the greats. Ben Johnson will never know if he could have beaten Carl Lewis that day at the Olympics. Tony Anderson will never know how it feels to play college football. Athletes who use drugs will always be asking, "How good could I have been if I hadn't used drugs?"

Financial Loss

Steve Howe says that he lost $5 million. He was highly paid, and he lost it all because he chose to use cocaine. Drug-using athletes can lose scholarships to college. There are high prices to be paid for drug use. Besides the potential money that is lost, buying drugs also costs a lot of money. The average steroid user spends from $50 to $600 every month, depending on the dosage. Marijuana users spend an average of $300 every month. Cocaine users spend between $60 and $120 for one tiny gram of cocaine. Crack users spend between $5 and $20 for each "rock" they buy, and crack addicts use many rocks every day. Drinking can also be a very expensive habit.

CHAPTER 5

Being the Best

Who is the best athlete you can think of? Who is the best hockey player? The best swimmer? The best tennis player? The best basketball player?

People will have different answers. The best hockey player might be Wayne Gretzky. The best swimmer might be Matt Biondi or Michael Gross. The best tennis player could be Stefi Graf.

Michael Jordan might be the best basketball player. He helped his college team win an NCAA championship. He won a gold medal in the 1984 Olympics. Since then, he has been playing for the Chicago Bulls. He was Rookie of the Year

47

48 his first season. He has set new NBA scoring records. He is a great offensive player and a great defensive player. He is the best player in the history of basketball, and he's just getting started.

One of the best swimmers in the world is Janet Evans. At the 1988 Olympics, she broke a world record in the 400-meter race. She also won three gold medals. She accomplished all that while she was still in high school.

Michael Jordan and Janet Evans are just two of the great athletes in the world. What makes them great? They have talent. They practice long, hard hours to be the best. They are also great because they are drug-free. They know that they can be the best without the use of drugs. They know that drugs would mess up their chances of being the very best they can be. Taking drugs would slow them down. It would affect their health. Top athletes stay on top by staying drug-free.

These athletes stay drug-free for other reasons, too. They know that they are role models. They have a responsibility to stay drug-free for the people who watch them compete. They know that they have to play fair and be good role models for themselves and for others.

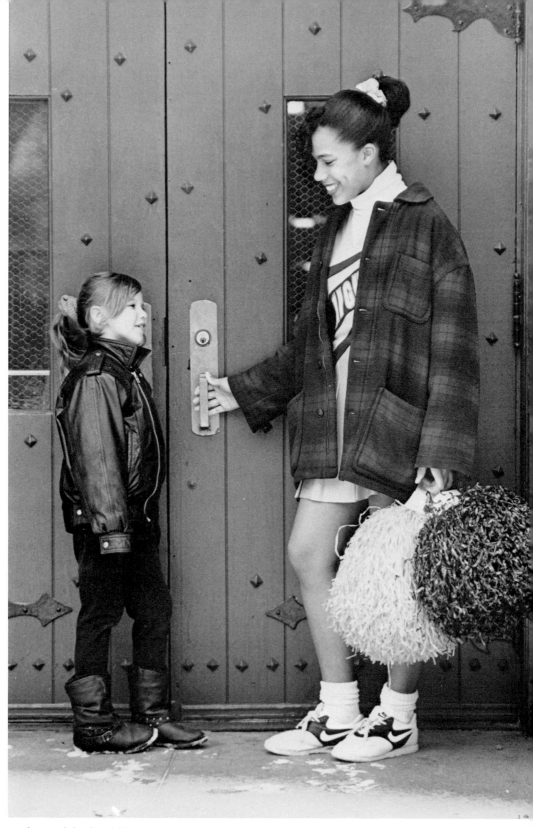

Role models should be good examples of discipline and determination for younger people.

50 | ## *Sports, Drugs, and You*

Since the beginning of time, people have been competing against each other. They compete to push each other to be better. They compete to test how far the human body can go. We want to achieve what other people can only dream of.

Today's athletes run faster than any others in history. They ski faster. They do difficult gymnastic stunts that were thought impossible 10 years ago. Every day athletes are proving that human beings are capable of amazing feats in sports.

People also compete with each other because it is fun. It's great to hear the roar of a crowd at any sporting event. It's fun to work with a team to prove that you are the best. It's fun to work up a sweat battling on a tennis court.

We want to feel the thrill of victory. We also want to learn how to lose with honor. Whether we win or lose, the thrill of great competition is always there.

Playing sports gives us so much. When we are chosen for a team we feel good about ourselves. We believe in our own talents. Even if we only play sports on the street or in school, it still feels good to be playing. Sports let us feel good about ourselves.

Sports also teach us discipline. To be good, you have to practice. You have to play by the rules and be healthy. You have to be willing to follow orders and work very hard. Mental and physical discipline are important to being a good athlete.

Being a good athlete also means choosing good role models. People like Michael Jordan and Janet Evans are good role models. They don't do drugs. They work hard, and they are the best. People like Len Bias and other drug users are bad role models. They are no longer the best at what they do. Choose good role models and try to follow their road to success.

When it comes to competition, you have to rely on your natural talents, not drugs. You can also make sure that all the competitors are playing fair. You can ask that drug testing be done.

You can also report it when someone on a team is using drugs. Tell your other teammates. Try to use positive peer pressure to get the user to stop. Ask the coach to talk to the team about drugs.

Nobody wants one drunk or stoned player to blow a game for the whole team. Nobody wants a teammate to be injured either. The game will be fair and fun only if every athlete is drug-free.

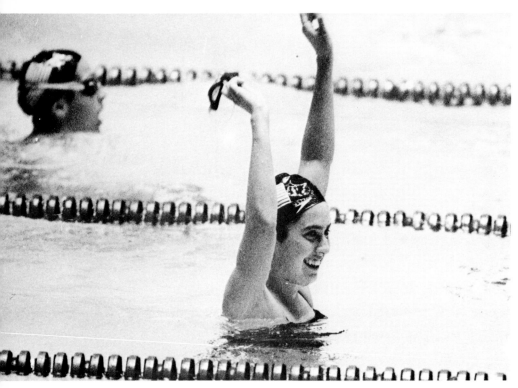

Janet Evans is a winner and a good role model because of hard work and determination.

What Can You Do?

To be a good athlete, there are some things you need to do. The most important thing is stay away from drugs.

You can ignore the people who offer the drugs. You can leave a party if drugs are present. You can tell your friends that you care about them, that you don't want to see them get messed up with drugs.

Use any method you feel comfortable with. If you say no often enough, they will stop offering it. As an athlete, you have a responsibility to say no. Your team counts on you. The fans count on you. Most of all, you owe it to yourself to be the best that you can be.

Set a good example. Be drug-free. You will inspire others to be drug-free, too.

If you suspect that someone is using drugs, you can look for some of these warning signs:

- Family problems
- Weight loss (cocaine, speed...)
- Weight gain (steroids, alcohol...)
- Shorter attention span
- Changing circle of friends
- Tardiness (showing up late)
- Money problems
- Depression
- Violent or aggressive actions
- Lying
- Lower performance (grades, sports...)
- Fatigue
- Red eyes
- Health problems

If someone you know has a problem with drugs, you can help. You can educate yourself about drug use in many ways. Read books about drugs. Watch television shows or news items about drug abuse. Ask your parents, teachers, and doctors about drugs. Talk to the minister at church or the local drug-abuse agency.

54 Once you have the information, try to pass it on to the drug-using person. Get a list of phone numbers that can be called for help. Be prepared to answer questions about drugs with the correct information.

Just telling a drug user about the bad effects will not do it all. A person with a drug problem needs help. Remember, it does not matter how often he or she uses drugs. What matters is what happens to him or her when using them. What happens to the people around him? That will tell you if the person has a problem. You need to talk to the person's parents. Don't ever worry about being a "narc." The parents have a right to know and help. Your friend will appreciate the help someday.

You can help the drug user by being concerned. You can show that you care. Ignoring the drug use will not help. Talk to the user only while he or she is sober.

Here are some guidelines for talking with a person about a drug problem.

- Be understanding. Listen to the person's reasons for using alcohol or other drugs.
- Be educated: Explain why you feel that use of alcohol or other drugs is

harmful and why you feel that the
person needs to seek counseling.

- Be supportive: Help the person find
  help and let him or her know that
  you will be there when needed in the
  tough times ahead.
- Be a good role model: Look at your
  own actions.

Approaching somebody about drug use
can be very difficult. You need to handle
the situation with care. The person will
usually deny that there is a problem. He
or she will try to put you on the defensive
by saying things like, "I thought that you
were my friend; are you calling me a drug
addict?" Stay calm and handle the
situation.

- Do not become emotional and argue
  about it.
- Do not make excuses for the person.
- Do not take over his or her duties to
  help.
- Do not try to talk sense while the person is drunk or high.
- Do not accept responsibility for the
  person's actions.
- Do not feel guilty for his or her drug-
  use problem.

Fact Sheet

- 3 million people have tried steroids.
- $100 million worth of steroids are sold every year.
- 60% of all crime is drug-related.
- Smoking is directly related to 400,000 deaths each year.
- One can of beer contains as much alcohol as one ounce of liquor.
- Diet pills are drugs (amphetamines).
- One police officer fighting drugs is killed every 57 hours.
- An estimated 30% of NFL players use steroids.
- Marijuana stays in the bloodstream for up to 30 days.
- First contact with drugs is usually through a friend.
- Marijuana today is 10–12 times more potent than the marijuana used in the 1960s.

- There are more than 10,000 antidrug clubs across the U.S.

- 80 brands of steroids are on the market.

- 1 in 15 high school seniors "admitted" using steroids.

- Drinking experience today usually starts around age 12.

- 25 million Americans have tried cocaine.

- Drug users make up the largest number of school dropouts.

- Crack is 10 times more powerful than cocaine.

- Murders in Washington, D.C., have doubled since crack appeared.

- Steroids cost between $50 and $600 per month depending on dosage.

- 93% of all people who have tried cocaine used marijuana first.

- Drug use is higher among those who have not finished high school.

Glossary
Explaining New Words

abuse Overuse of drugs in illegal or unsafe ways.

aggressive Quick to attack others.

Al-Anon Group of people who have chemically dependent family members; they meet to help each other.

Alateen Group like Al-Anon for young people.

alcoholics People who have a disease called alcoholism; they are dependent on alcohol.

Alcoholics Anonymous Group of alcoholics who meet regularly to help one another stay well.

alcoholism Illness that causes people to become dependent on alcohol.

chemical dependence Illness that occurs when someone is mentally or physically dependent on a drug.

cirrhosis Disease of the liver that can be caused by heavy drinking.

cocaine Powerful stimulant.

crack Extremely powerful, smokable form of cocaine.

drug Any substance other than food or water which, when taken into the body, changes how the mind or body works.

drug addict Person who is dependent on a drug other than alcohol.

experimentation Use of drugs to find out how they will affect you.

gateway drugs Drugs that lead to the use of harder drugs. Tobacco, alcohol, and marijuana are gateway drugs.

hallucinations Seeing, hearing, or feeling things that are not real.

marijuana Plant that is illegal to grow, sell, buy, or use because of the drug it contains.

nervous system The brain, spinal cord, and nerves.

nicotine The stimulant in tobacco that can cause dependency.

overdose Enough of a drug to cause illness or death.

peers People your own age.

prescription Note a doctor writes to a pharmacist ordering a medicine.

recover To become well.

self-confidence Belief in your own abilities.

self-esteem How you view or feel about yourself.

symptoms Changes in your body indicating that you have a disease.

tar Sticky, brown substance found in tobacco.

Help List

Alcohol Hotline:
800-ALCOHOL (252-6465)

Al-Anon (for families of alcoholics):
800-344-2666

Narcotics Anonymous:
818-780-3951

Nar-Anon (for families of drug users)
213-547-5800

Cocaine Hotline:
800-COCAINE (262-2463)

National Institute on Drug Abuse
(Prevention Branch):
800-638-2045

NIDA Help Line:
800-622-HELP

"Just Say NO" Hotline:
800-258-2766

Secret Witness Hotline (to report drug activity):
800-732-7463

You may also want to write for information. Many organizations will send you free information if you ask.

Al-Anon/Alateen Family Group Headquarters:
P.O. Box 862, Midtown Station
New York, NY 10018

American Council for Drug Education
204 Monroe Street
Rockville, MD 20850

COCANON:
P.O. Box 64742-66
Los Angeles, CA 90064

Institute on Black Chemical Abuse:
2616 Nicollet Avenue
Minneapolis, MN 55408

Nar-Anon Family Group Headquarters:
P.O. Box 2562
Palos Verdes Peninsula, CA 92704

National Association for Children of Alcoholics:
31706 Coast Highway
South Laguna, CA 92677

For Further Reading

Berger, Gilda. *Making Up Your Mind about Drugs*. New York: Lodestar Books, 1988.

Peck, Rodney. *Crack*. New York: Rosen Publishing Group, 1991.

Scott, Sharon. *How to Say No and Keep Your Friends*. Amherst, MA: Human Resource Development Press, 1986.

———. *When to Say Yes and Make More Friends*. Amherst, MA: Human Resource Development Press, 1988.

Seixas, Judith S. *Alcohol—What It Is, What It Does*. New York: Greenwillow Books, 1977.

———. *Tobacco—What It Is, What It Does*. New York: Greenwillow Books, 1981.

Taylor, Barbara. *Everything You Need to Know about Alcohol*. New York: Rosen Publishing Group, 1989.

Not as easy to read, but worth looking at:

Gold, Mark. *The Facts about Drugs and Alcohol*. New York: Bantam Books, 1988.

———. *800-COCAINE*. New York: Bantam Books, 1988.

Harris, Jonathan. *Drugged Athletes: The Crisis in America*. New York: Four Winds Press, 1987.

Index

About the Author

Rodney Peck is a graduate of Central Michigan University. It was at Central Michigan that he became involved with the America's PRIDE program. The program uses attractive alternatives such as dancing, singing, acting, and speaking as ways to combat drug use. Peck worked and performed with the National PRIDE team for four years. He has spoken to thousands of young people on the topics of peer pressure, self-esteem, and drug use. Currently he is a Peace Corps Volunteer working in drug education in Belize, Central America.

Photo Credits

Cover Photo: Stuart Rabinowitz
Photos on pages 2, 6, 14, 17, 18, 23, 28, 32, 38, 49: Dru Nadler; pages 11, 31: Chris Volpe; page 35: Jill Heisler Jacks; pages 43, 52: AP/Wide World Photos.

Design & Production: Blackbirch Graphics, Inc